Periods Around the World: People, Places, and Perspectives

Pia Apurva, Kyli Chu, Eloise Hamilton, Anya Peterson, Serena Saleih, and Divya Subramanian

Edited by: Kristen Gianaris, Paula Araque, and Sameeksha Singh

Illustrated by: Sadie Chou

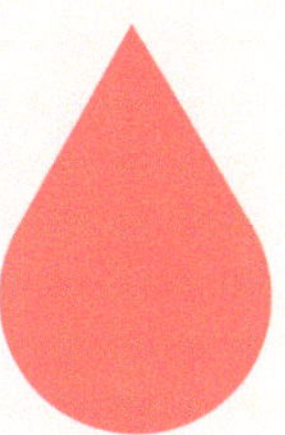

Introduction

Hello! If you picked up this book, you might be interested in learning more about menstruation and period cultures around the world. Well, you're in luck! After receiving a grant from the City of Seattle and working with our global studies teacher to identify a social issue that was important to us, we (a group of eighth-grade students) decided to explore the topic of menstrual health. As people who experience periods, we are keen to learn more about this process and how it impacts people differently around the world. In this book, we hope to teach you a bit about what periods are, the traditions and cultures that influence the diverse experiences that people with periods have, and the various perspectives attached to this natural cycle. We will also highlight a few impressive change-makers and leaders around the world who are advocating for an end to period poverty, more accessibility surrounding products and education, and destigmatization.

Periods happen to people who have a uterus—regardless of their gender identity. Menarche, the first menstrual cycle, most commonly occurs between the ages of 10 and 15 but can happen earlier or later depending on when a person begins puberty. Getting a period for the first time is central to both social and medical perspectives of growth and development all around the world. Although not all people with periods are able to have biological children, getting a period introduces the possibility of fertility. Puberty, including menarche, results from a shift in hormones, such as estrogen and progesterone.

These hormones are responsible for the body's hair growth, muscle development, voice changes, breast development, shifts in the reproductive tract, mood changes, sleep cycles, stress management, and more. Not only do these hormones change significantly during puberty, but they also change during each monthly menstrual cycle.

When people with ovaries reach a certain age—usually between forty-five and fifty-five—their body goes through a process called "menopause," which is another major hormonal shift. This means that they'll stop experiencing their period for good and will no longer be fertile.

Many people with a uterus are sensitive to the fluctuations in hormones. These sensitivities can cause people with a period to experience pain, mood disorders, heavy bleeding, and a number of other complications or challenging experiences throughout the menstrual cycle.

Sadly, due to a lack of research and funding related to menstrual health and experiences, menstruating people are not properly understood, and they are often mistreated by medical practitioners. In fact, there are many taboos and stigmas surrounding the menstrual process, which can make it difficult to openly discuss these relevant issues and experiences with others. However, getting a period is a natural process and is even celebrated in some communities and cultures.

Throughout history, perspectives on the menstrual process have shifted. Here, we urge a worldwide shift toward acceptance, education, understanding, care, and compassion regarding menstrual health and the cultures attached to it. Let's learn from each other and share our stories!

It's important to recognize that it would be impossible for us to cover the full range of experiences and cultural beliefs related to menstruation. Our goal, simply put, is to share a few stories, anecdotes, facts, and experiences related to periods around the world. The information written in this book is based on the interviews that we conducted with people from our global community. Additionally, we carried out research and shared our own experiences related to menstrual health. Most of the people we interviewed expressed concerns about the taboos associated with period culture and the challenges associated with menstruating. Their common desires included establishing equitable access to sex education, building support systems, and exploring options of paid menstrual leave.

What is a period?

A period, also known as a part of the menstrual cycle, is the monthly shedding of the uterus lining. The shedding causes a combination of blood and tissue to flow from the uterus through the cervix and out of the vagina. Although most people's cycles vary slightly in terms of duration, side effects, and overall experience, the process remains the same. The purpose of this process is to prepare the body for a potential pregnancy.

The average cycle is 28 days; however, a normal cycle for some people could be anywhere between 23-35 days. A cycle begins the day one gets their period (starts menstrual bleeding) and ends the day their next period starts.

The Reproductive Tract

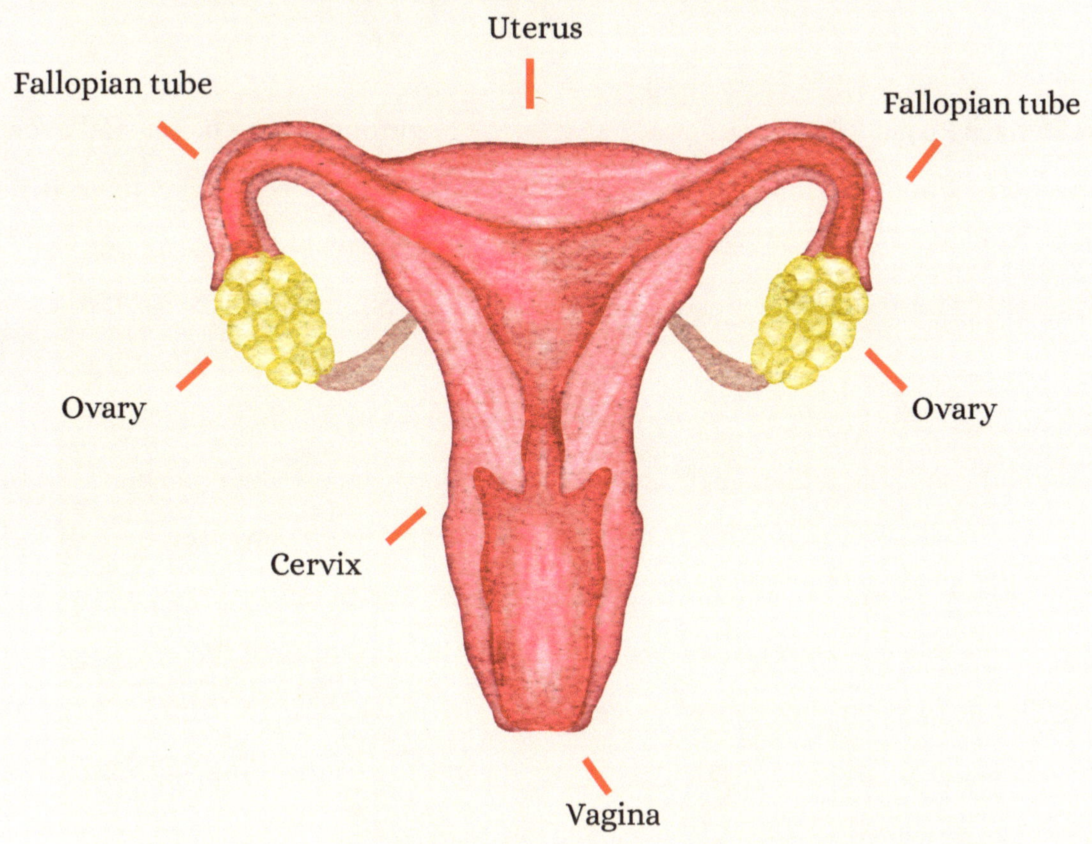

The Four Phases of the Menstrual Cycle

1) The Menses Phase: The menses phase marks the beginning of the menstrual cycle. This is when a period/menstrual bleeding commences. Menstrual bleeding usually lasts between three to seven days. Menstruation is driven by chemical messengers in your body called "hormones." These alert the uterus to either shed its lining or prepare itself to reproduce.

2) The Follicular Phase: Typically taking place between days six and fourteen of the menstrual cycle, the follicular phase is when levels of the estrogen hormone rise in the body. The level of estrogen in a person's body affects their reproductive tract, urinary tract, skin, hair, mucous membranes, bones, heart and blood vessels, and brain. Most estrogen is produced in the ovaries, although small amounts of the hormone are also created by the adrenal glands and fat cells. This process causes the lining of the uterus to thicken in order to prepare for an egg to implant in the uterus lining, if pregnancy were to occur.

3) The Ovulation Phase: During ovulation, the luteinizing hormone is released, triggering the ovaries to release an egg. Ovulation is the fertile time of the cycle, becoming a moment to keep track of when planning for or avoiding a pregnancy. Ovulation typically happens twelve to fourteen days after the first day of your menstrual cycle. If the egg is fertilized by a sperm during sex, pregnancy occurs. If there is no fertilization, the uterus prepares to shed blood and tissue for another round of menstrual bleeding.

4) The Luteal Phase: During the luteal phase (typically between days fifteen and twenty-eight), the egg leaves the ovary and begins its journey through the fallopian tubes and into the uterus. The level of the hormone progesterone rises during this time. Like estrogen (which begins to decrease during this phase), progesterone helps to prepare the uterine lining for a potential pregnancy. It is also responsible for regulating moods, supporting thyroid function, regulating sleep, and more. An increase in progesterone can cause symptoms such as bloating, breast tenderness and swelling, anxiety or agitation, fatigue, weight gain, and a shift in overall mood.

EUPHEMISMS FOR MENSTRUATION AROUND THE WORLD

PERIOD · AUNT FLO · ON THE RAG · CHECKING INTO THE RED ROOF INN · LADY BUSINESS · THAT TIME OF THE MONTH · MOON TIME · SHARK WEEK · CRIMSON TIDE · BLUE DAY · LITTLE RED · OLD FRIEND · RED ARMY · CRITICAL DAYS · THE RULE · THE PAINTER IN THE STAIRWAY · I FEEL SICK · STRAWBERRY SEASON · I HAVE A FLOOD · THE MONSTER · MY ELDEST AUNT · MY RELATIVES · THE MONTHLY THING · GIRL STUFF · I AM BROKEN · THE RED SEA · MY MOON · RED WEEK · CHUMS · YOUR DEVILS · MY GOOD FRIEND · THE THING · THE LADY IN RED · MY BLEED · MOTHER NATURE'S GIFT · CODE RED

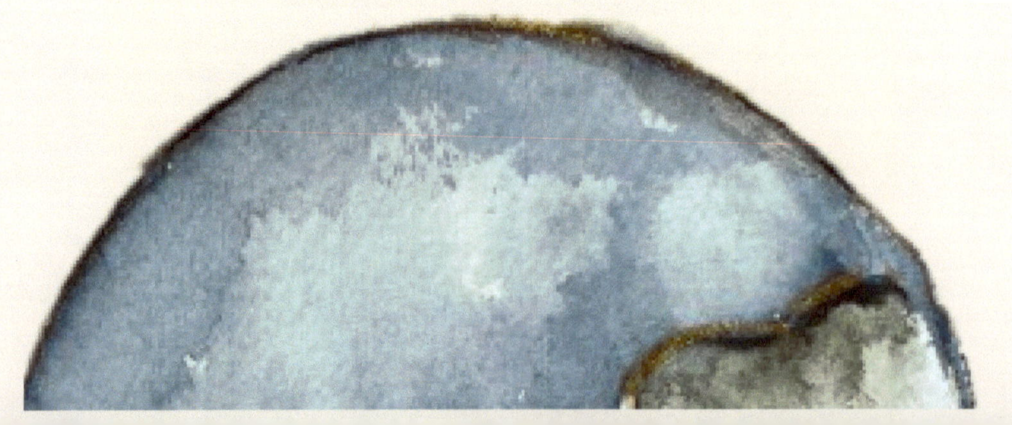

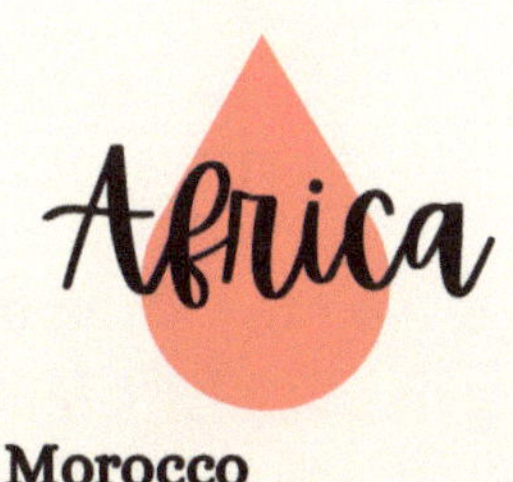

Africa

Morocco

Along with ninety-nine percent of Morocco's population, Aicha practices Islam. During the holy month of Ramadan, Muslims fast from sunrise to sunset. However, when a woman is on her period, she is not required to fast. Still, it's socially unacceptable to eat or drink in front of others, so when Aicha was young, her grandmother scolded her for drinking tisanes (an herbal remedy to ease aches and pains) in front of her uncles during Ramadan. As Aicha grows older, she better understands the taboos associated with menstruation. However, she is eager to normalize conversations around periods and create safe spaces for others to share their experiences.

Kenya

In 2004, Kenya became the first country in the world to eliminate taxes on tampons. Advocates against period poverty are pushing for free access to menstrual supplies across the country. Kenyan senator, Gloria Orwoba, is working to eradicate stigmas about periods by encouraging men to talk about them and campaigning to end period shaming. In 2023, Senator Orwoba was asked to leave the parliament building over a "period stain" on her pants. She is behind a motion that increases period funding and addresses period poverty.

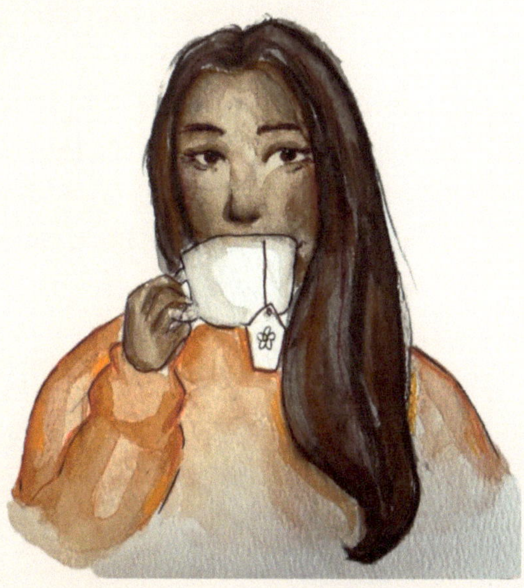

Egypt

According to a 2018 study conducted by the Middle East Fertility Society Journal in Beni-Suef, a city in Northern Egypt, 92% of women experience dysmenorrhea (painful cramps) during their period, and 86.3% experience symptoms of PMS (premenstrual syndrome). This is not unique to Egypt. In fact, around the world, at least 90% of people with a uterus report symptoms of PMS.

Ethiopia

Samrawit is from Ethiopia, which is a part of the Horn of Africa. In one of Ethiopa's national languages, Amharic, menstruation is called *"yewor abeba,"* meaning "monthly flower." The metaphor stems from the idea that flowering plants usually produce fruit, the same way that periods offer the possibility of fertility, or producing life.

Samrawit experiences premenstrual dysphoric disorder (PMDD) and wishes that her peers and teachers would discuss it more. Similar to PMS, PMDD causes Samrawit to feel changes in her behavior and emotions more severely than others. PMDD is extremely prevalent in Ethiopia and many other countries. It can heavily affect a person experiencing it. Today, Samrawit shares her experiences with PMDD to help others become more aware of what it is and how to treat it.

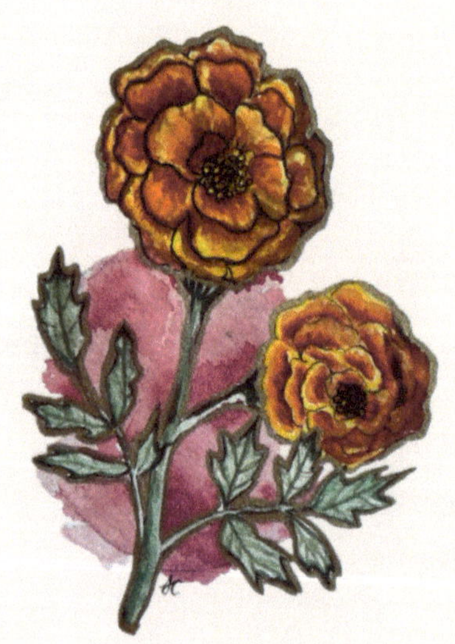

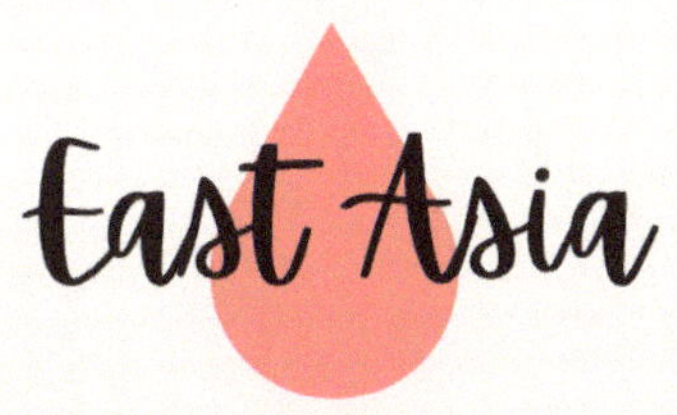

East Asia

China

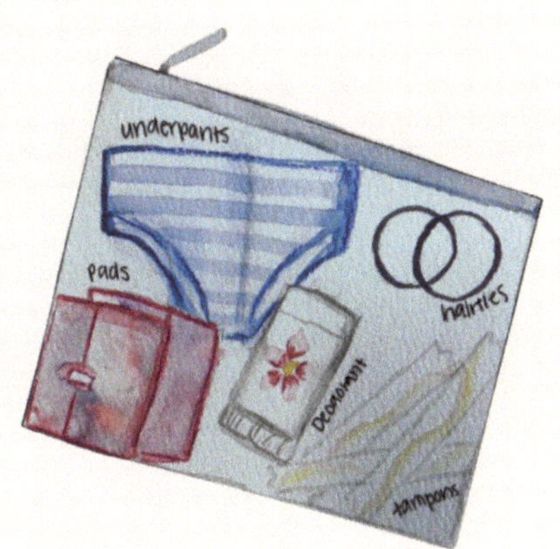

When Mei got her period, she didn't understand what was happening. Since the topic of menstruation wasn't commonly discussed in her communities, she hadn't even talked to her mother or sisters about the experience. She remembers coming home from school that day and whispering to her mother that she was given pads by her teacher. One day, while Mei was on her period, her family was going to visit a temple, but they told her she couldn't come because she was menstruating. Mei wasn't allowed into temples to worship or gravesites to visit ancestors, because menstruating was considered "dirty" and going into a temple or gravesite would make it "impure."

Japan

In Sakura's history class, she read about the 1928
Tokyo Municipal Bus Company strikes and post-
World War II strikes, which were led by women
who struggled with the lack of sanitary facilities
and accommodations in workplaces. Finally, in
1947, Japan introduced menstrual leave in the
country's labor laws. This new law entitled
women to days off of work while on their period.

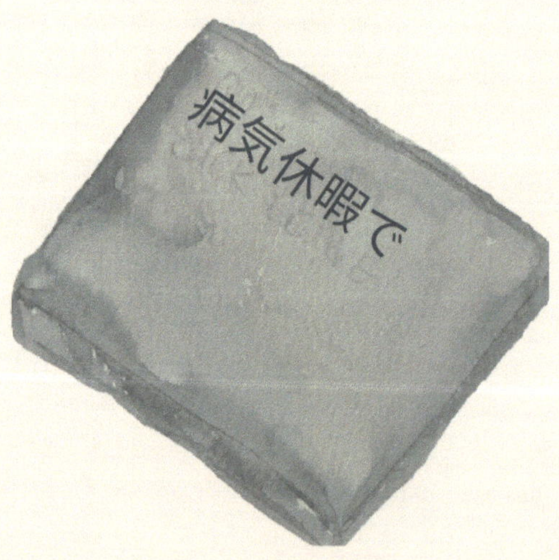

South Korea

When Hyo got their period, their mom made Patjuk (red bean porridge), a traditional comfort food in Korea made with rice and red beans. Patjuk is eaten during special times of the year, such as the winter solstice. The food is said to help ward off bad spirits and unfortunate luck.

Despite South Korea being a country where discussing periods is widely considered taboo, the capital city, Seoul, opened its first "Period Shop" in 2021. The Period Shop is dedicated to creating opportunities for customers to openly explore and purchase menstrual supplies. It emphasizes sustainability by working to eradicate waste that comes with many period products. According to South Korea's Ministry of Food and Drug Safety, more than 81% of women used disposable sanitary pads during their period in 2017. In addition to a variety of menstrual products, the shop also sells items that might relieve stress and pain throughout the menstrual cycle.

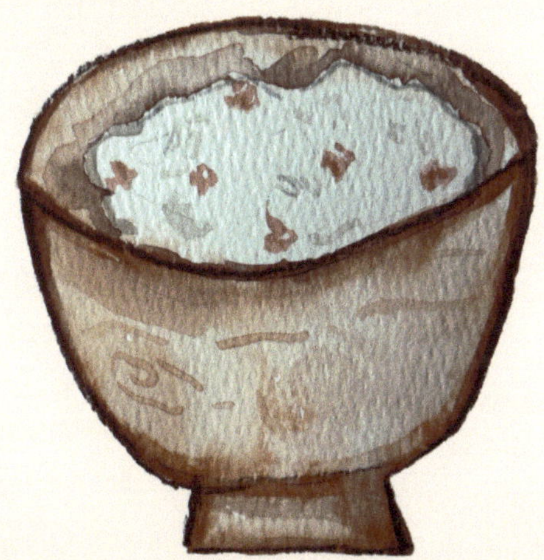

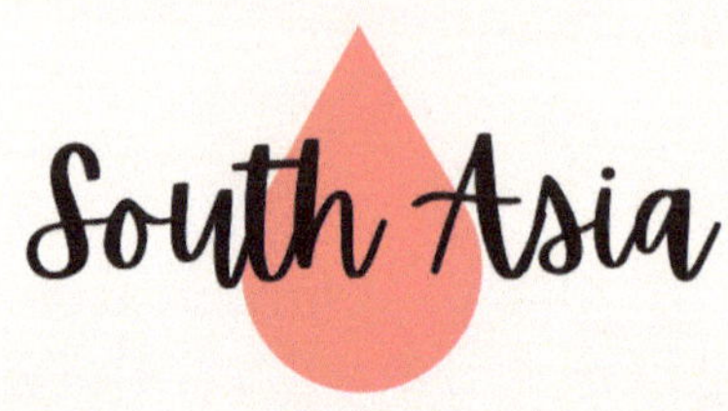

South Asia

India

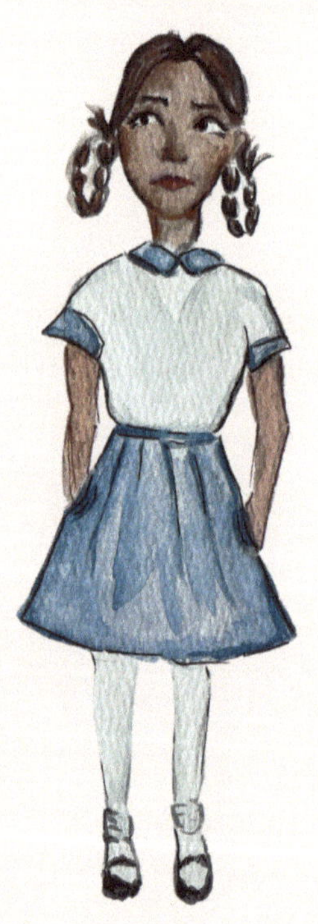

In India, some people refer to their periods as "chums." When Shriya first got her period, her mother told her that she had come of age. Her grandmother gave her a necklace and congratulated her on having grown up! Her family informed her that from then on, she would not be able to enter the temple or prayer room during her menstruation. Her mother also told her to be careful around sacred plants so that their energy wouldn't be affected. Since it is taboo to talk about periods in India, Shriya was cautioned not to talk about her "chums" with others. These traditions are common among Hindu communities in India. It is often speculated that such practices come from the Hindu mythological story of Indra's slaying of Vritra, the connection being that menstruating people were taking on portions of Indra's guilt that came from Vritra's death.

When Aliyah first got her period, she was eleven years old. When her periods began to cause excruciating pain, she learned that she had endometriosis, a condition in which tissue grows on the outside of the uterus. Among others, the symptoms of endometriosis include cramps, painful bowel movements, urination during a period, fertility issues, heavy period flows, digestive problems, painful sexual intercourse, and fatigue. Unfortunately, Aliyah is not the only one experiencing this in her home country; Afghanistan has the second-highest rate of reported endometriosis worldwide.

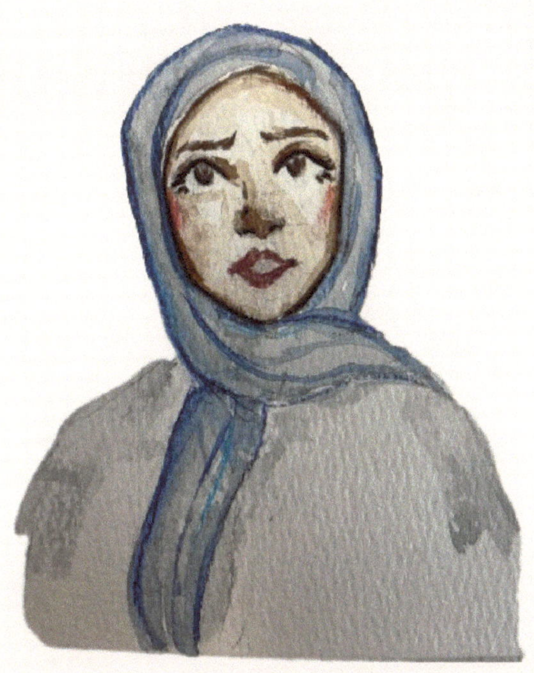

Pakistan

Growing up, Ayesha did not receive much education about puberty and menstrual cycles. In fact, it is estimated that approximately 50% of women in Pakistan receive little to no information about periods before their first menstrual cycle. Being differently abled, Ayesha struggled at times to access menstrual products. However, that changed in 2018 when activist Tanzila Khan created a mobile app called *"Girlythings."* The app offers a delivery service for those who are unable to access stores that sell period products. It also serves as a platform to promote inclusivity and educational resources surrounding menstruation.

Sri Lanka

When Bhagya got her first period, her grandma told her it was a cause for celebration. She mentioned that her family would call a priest to perform a rite where she would undergo the holy, symbolic ritual of being bathed or sprinkled in saffron and milk. She would also wear a sari for the very first time. This completed her entrance into womanhood.

Oceania

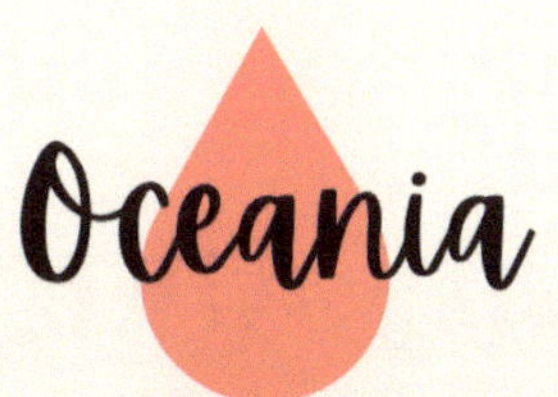

Australia

Beau lives in Australia, and when they got their period, they were excited to use the phrases their mom had taught them. They told their friends that they were on "shark week" and that "the painters were in the hallway." Beau loves learning, so when they discovered that the most popular pad brand in Australia had fun facts on the packaging, they were more than excited! The facts ranged from animals to history and were often a reason to look forward to their "shark week."

Aboriginal and Indigenous Australians

Kaiya is an Indigenous Australian. When she got her period, she was provided with many of the resources she needed; however, many of her relatives and friends struggled to get access to period products. The price of menstruation products is skyrocketing and becoming unaffordable. When Kaiya grew up, she knew she had to help combat this issue, so she joined an organization called "Share the Dignity." This organization helps provide menstruation resources to support Indigenous Australians as well as others who need them.

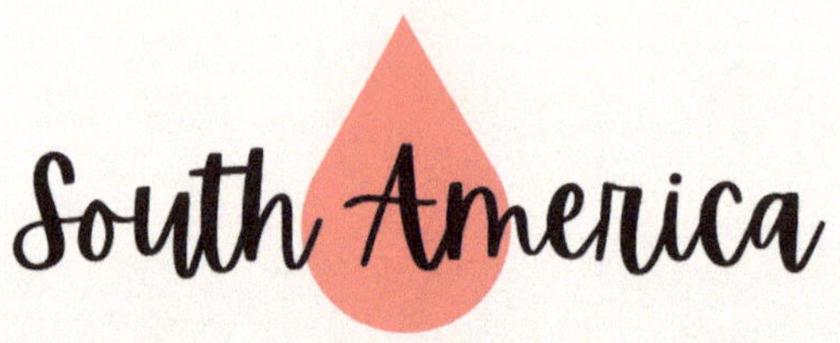

Colombia

When Mariana got her period in Colombia, her mom congratulated her and gave her a book called *Cosas de Niña*, which translates to "Girl Stuff." The book taught her what to do when she got her period and how to deal with issues that could come up. Although the book was helpful, she was still left with many questions. As she grew up, she realized that not everyone in her country could openly talk about their period, even with their family. She grew increasingly passionate about this issue, so she joined the fight for period awareness in Colombia.

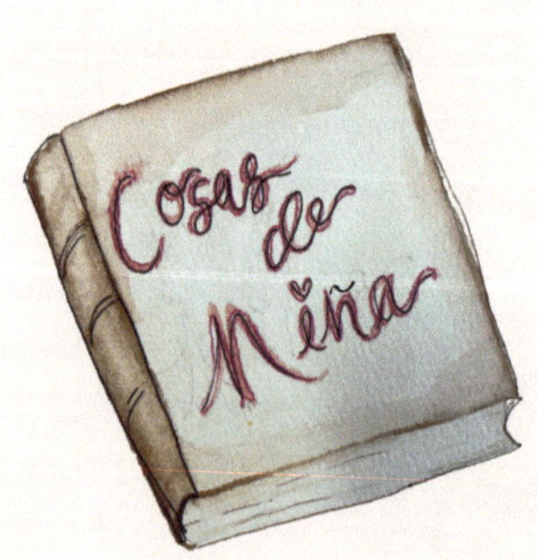

Amazonian Ticuna

Matilde lives in Brazil. She is part of the Amazonian Ticuna, an indigenous people native to Brazil, Peru, and Colombia. When Matilde got her first period, she was instructed to stay alone in a special room. During this time, the elder women in her community would visit her, sharing aspects of their culture and traditions. She learned songs, myths, and stories passed on from generations. For Matilde, her time in isolation lasted two weeks, but for some people, it can last up to six months. When Matilde finished her isolation, Pelazón commenced. Pelazón is a four-day celebration that commemorates coming of age and womanhood. The ceremony includes fire, singing, and dancing. Matilde was taken to the water on the last day and placed alongside a newborn. This step of the ceremony is considered the final cleansing before Matilde becomes an adult.

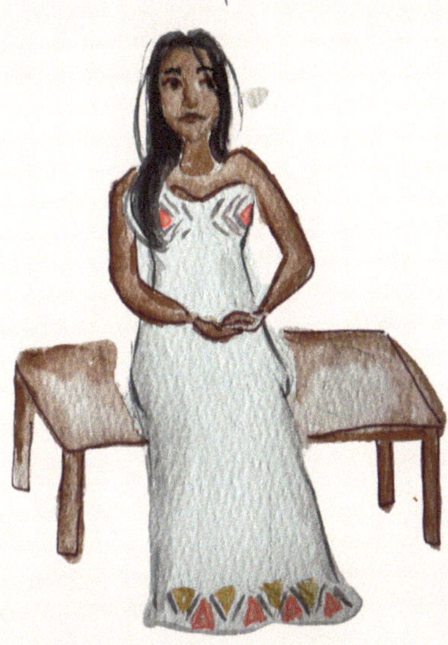

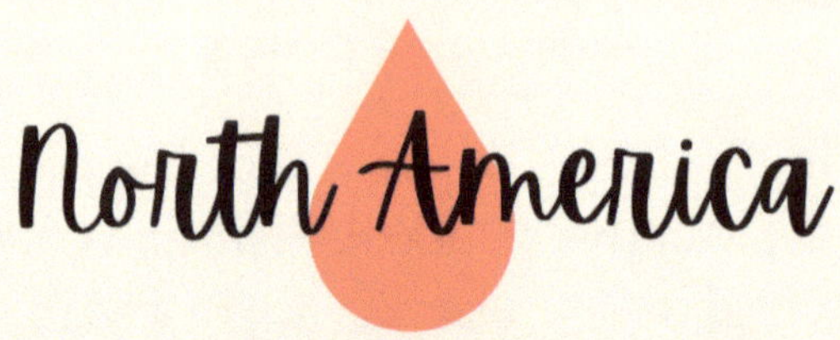

North America

The United States

In the United States, there are different laws and regulations surrounding sex education, including discussions about menstrual health, depending on which state one resides in. Suzy grew up in Washington State where schools are required to teach comprehensive sex education. In fifth grade she took a "Family Life and Sexual Health" class, and in seventh grade she took a "Gender Studies" class. However, in states such as Florida, sex education is not required and young people tend to have less access to formal sex education.

Lakota Nation

Many Lakota people across North America celebrate periods—especially a person's menarche—as a powerful time to purify one's body. The menstrual process can be spiritual and may strengthen a sense of community among women.

Kimimela was very excited when she got her period, otherwise known as her "moon time," because when she is on her moon time, she is considered to be very powerful and strong. In fact, the women in her tribe are considered very sacred as they are life-givers. They cannot touch medicinal plants because they could draw away their energy. In the past, Kimimela's ancestors used parts of the cedar tree instead of pads.

Mexico

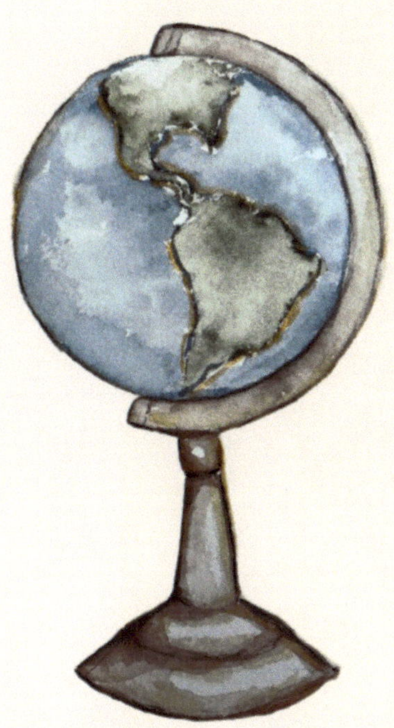

Maria recalls the first time her grandmother taught her about what some of her friends called her "regalo." Regalo, meaning "gift" in Spanish, sounds similar to the word "regla," meaning menstruation. At the age of twelve, when her *gift* finally came, her grandmother celebrated by preparing an aromatic bath, lighting a candle, and encouraging Maria to rest. She told Maria, "Your body is now a woman, but your heart is still childlike." She whispered prayers while she anointed her and made reusable pads in an effort to protect the environment from the waste of disposable ones. Maria wasn't allowed to bathe for the following days of her period, and she was instructed to avoid eating sour foods and sudden temperature changes. Her grandmother's approach to celebrating menarche stems from the histories and traditions of the Zapotec people from Southern Mexico.

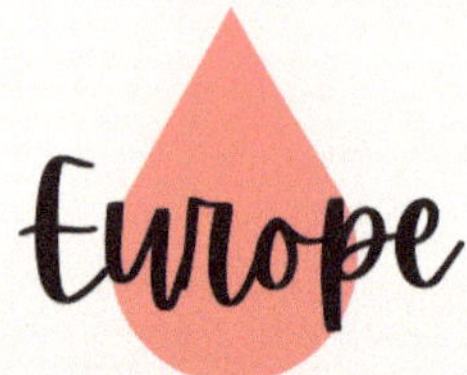

Europe

Italy

When Francesca got her period, the news spread far and wide. Everyone began calling her "signorina," which means "miss" or "young lady." This signified a rite of passage into adulthood. As everyone celebrated, her mother and older sister took her aside to explain all that this next phase in life entailed.

France

Ariel is Jewish and follows traditional beliefs that were formed through her understanding of the Torah. After she was married, she began observing a practice that required her to practice sexual abstinence during her *Niddah* (the Hebrew word for "menstruation") and the seven days following. On the seventh day after she stops bleeding each month, she dips into a *mikvah*. The word "mikvah" comes from the Hebrew word for "collection." It refers to a collection of water—especially natural water such as the ocean, a lake, or a large bathtub. The mikvah is a purification ritual that dates back thousands of years and is considered a powerful spiritual experience that symbolizes renewal and rejuvenation.

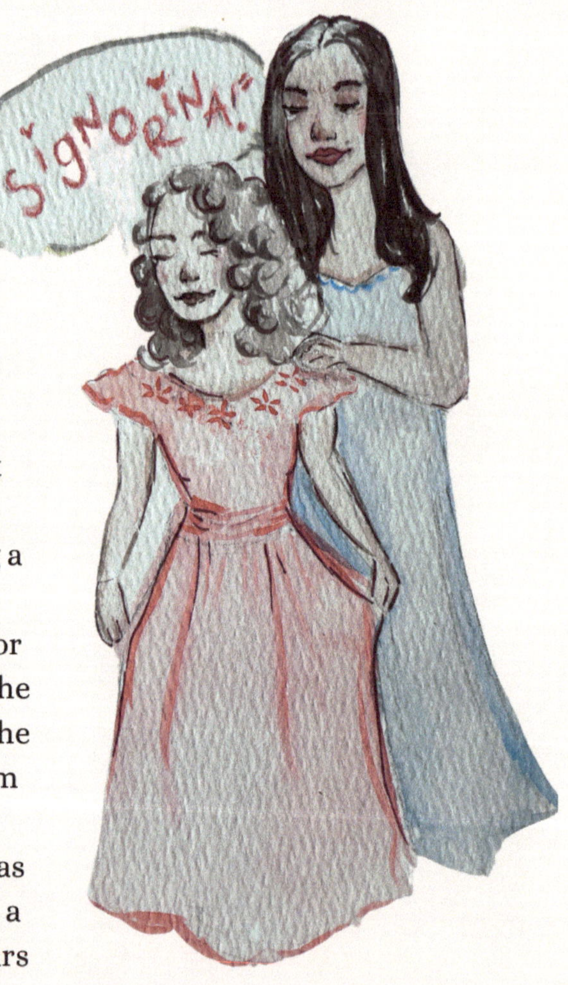

Germany

In Germany, Max referred to their period as "their bleed." When Max got their period, their family congratulated them and said, "The lady in red is coming!" They had already learned about periods in school with their classmates. Every Wednesday, Max had a class about sex education because it was valued just as much as other school subjects. It is a class that everyone has to take because it covers menstruation and reproductive health.

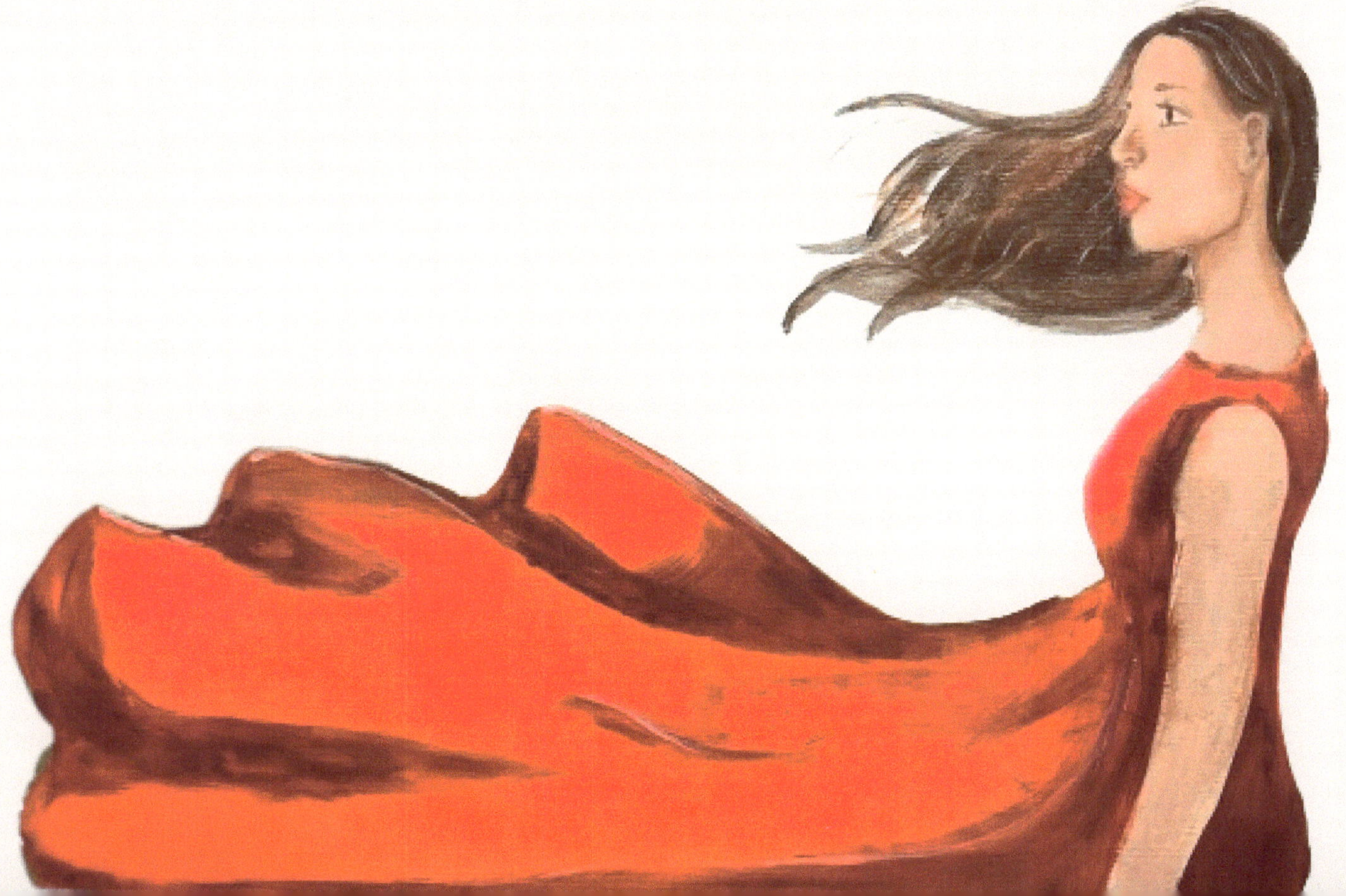

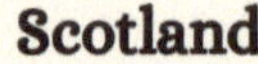

Scotland

In Scotland, when Eleanor first got her period, her mom made a cake and gave her a necklace to remember the special day. She enjoyed the cake with her family and wore her special necklace for the rest of the week. In 2020, Eleanor celebrated Scotland's decision to make period products free for anyone who needs them!

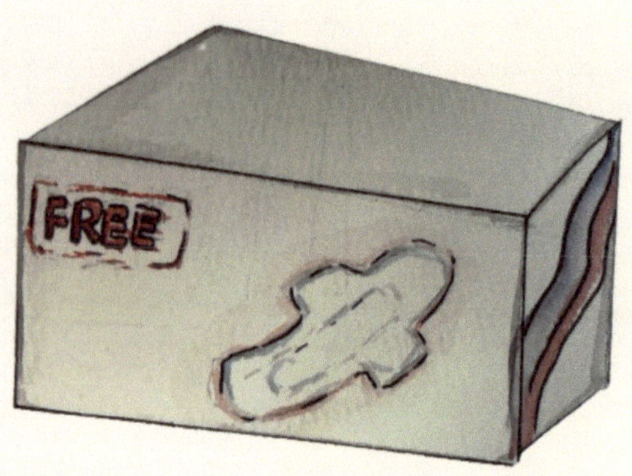

Spain

As of February 2023, Spain became the first country in the world to offer paid menstrual leave from work for up to five days. It makes sense; people with periods often have aches, cramps, or discomfort that accompanies their period. This law was created to help minimize taboos, normalize the conversation around periods, and allow for rest and recovery.

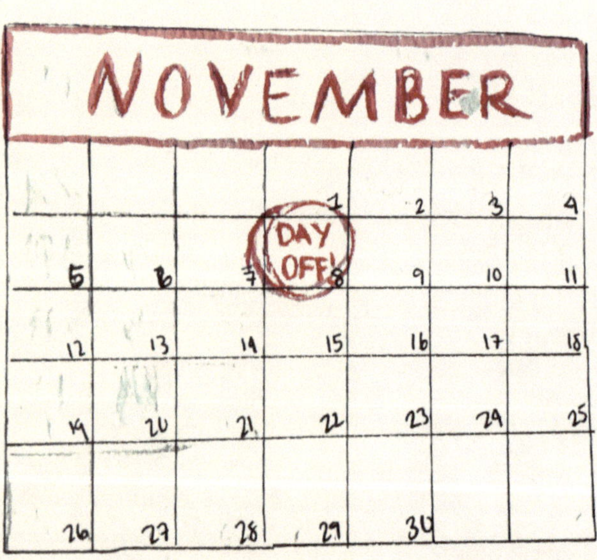

Related Terms Glossary

Adenomyosis: A condition in which the uterine lining begins to expand into the muscular walls of the uterus.

Birth Control: Refers to any method used to prevent pregnancy. Some methods include medications (e.g. pills and shots), medical procedures (e.g. sterilization), devices (e.g. condoms and intrauterine devices), and behaviors (e.g. abstinence and menstrual cycle tracking).

Endometriosis: A condition in which tissue that resembles the uterine lining grows outside of the uterus, causing painful periods and complications when trying to get pregnant.

Dysmenorrhea: The clinical term used to describe menstrual cramps. Some causes of dysmenorrhea include endometriosis, uterine fibroids, and adenomyosis.

Fertility: A person's ability to conceive children.

Hormones: Chemical messengers that send signals to different parts of your body to regulate physiology and behavior. Some hormones associated with menstrual cycles include progesterone, luteinizing hormone, and estrogen.

Menarche: Refers to the first time a person gets their period, marking the beginning of their menstrual cycle.

Menopause: Term used to refer to the period of twelve months after a person's last menstruation. Menopause involves the decline in reproductive hormones, causing the end of the menstrual cycle in a person's life. Menopausal symptoms include hot flashes, vaginal dryness, anxiety, and depression.

Menorrhagia: Also known as "having a heavy flow," menorrhagia is a condition in which menstruating people experience heavy or prolonged menstrual bleeding, causing side effects such as fatigue and shortness of breath.

Premenstrual Dysphoric Disorder (PMDD): A severe version of premenstrual syndrome (PMS), causing drastic physical and behavioral symptoms the week or two before the first day of menstruation. Symptoms include extreme mood shifts, tender breasts, and bloating.

Premenstrual Syndrome (PMS): Physical and behavioral changes that take place a week or two before the onset of menstruation. Symptoms include irritability, fatigue, changes in appetite, bloating, and mood swings.

Uterus: The organ in which offspring are conceived and where they gestate until birth. During the menstrual cycle, the uterus develops a lining to prepare for pregnancy. However, if no pregnancy occurs, then the lining is shed as a menstrual period.

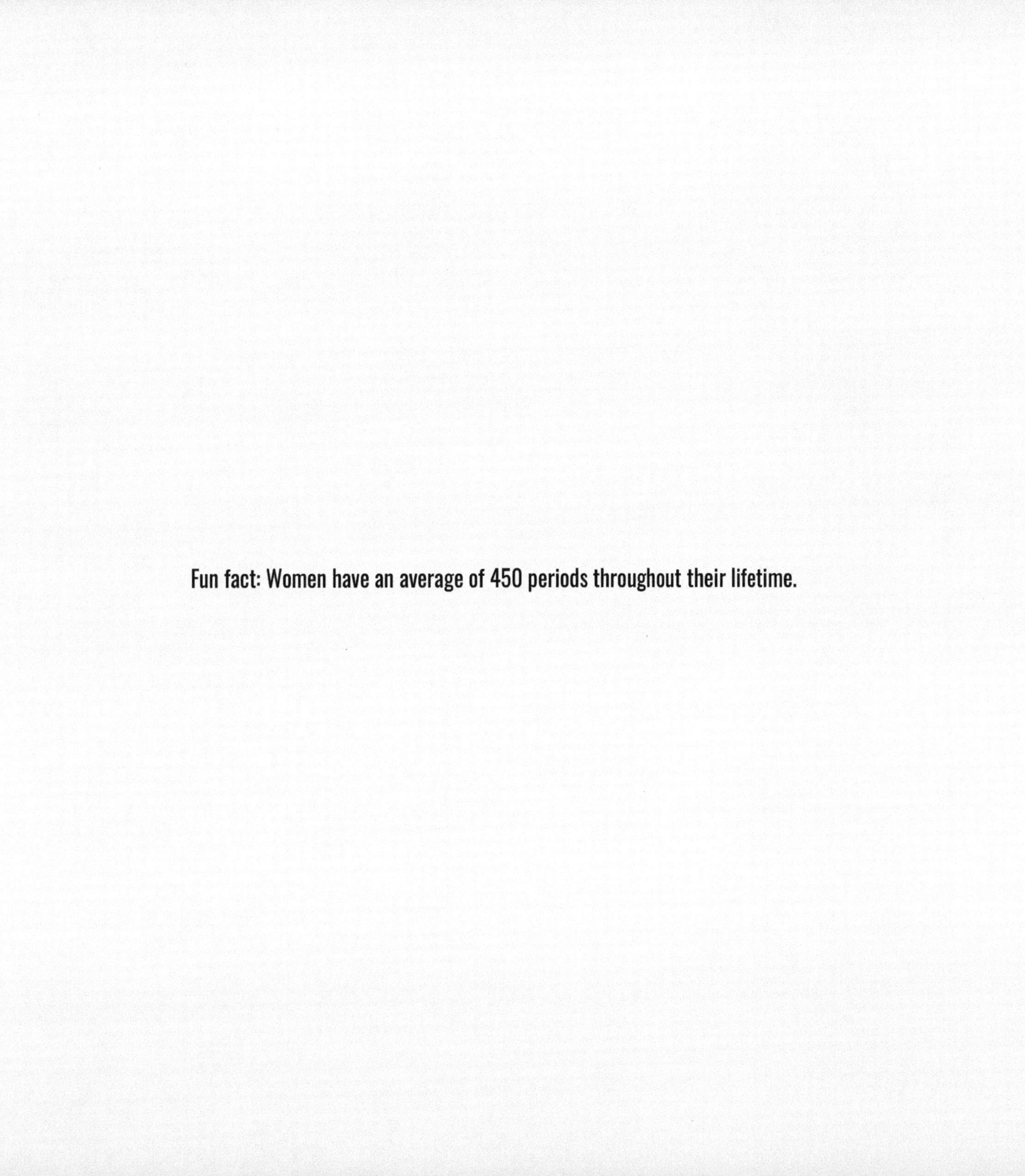

Fun fact: Women have an average of 450 periods throughout their lifetime.

Share your period story...

In an effort to document the wide variety of period stories around the world, celebrate our bodies, give attention to our natural cycles, encourage acceptance and understanding, and urge further medical research/education surrounding menstrual health for all people with a uterus, we hope that you will take the time to write your period story and even share it with others!

Share your story with us on Instagram: @periodsaroundtheworld

Acknowledgements

This project took a great amount of passion, dedication, and collaboration. We would not have been able to do it without our outstanding editors and teachers, Kristen Gianaris and Paula Araque, our student editor, Sameeksha Singh, and our incredibly talented illustrator, Sadie Chou.

We are beyond grateful that we had the opportunity to interview people with periods from around the world. We would specifically like to thank Elizabeth Dimond, Leila Benkassaoui, Kea Stieber, Rachel Johnson, Laura Bolan, Doris Koo, Lily Kim, Loyce Ong'udi, Charlie Ogilvie, Kim Nguyen, and Sandra Duarte. It has been an honor to learn from each one of you.

Meet the Authors

Anya Peterson: Anya loves to spend time with her family and friends playing games, eating food, reading books, and watching movies. In her free time, Anya also loves to play soccer, sing, and do art. She hopes to be an entrepreneur in the future and has loved getting to work on this project.

Divya Subramanian: Divya is a fun-loving individual who enjoys reading, music, and basketball. She can often be found reading a good book, playing her favorite tunes on the piano (entirely by ear), or shooting three-pointers outside. When she's not in school or pursuing her hobbies, Divya loves to spend time with friends and family, especially her amazing younger sister.

Eloise Hamilton: Eloise loves music, movies, friends, and family. She has two dogs named Lucy and Dixie. She loves to play basketball, do gymnastics, have fun with her teammates, and spend her free time with her friends. She also loves to bake and eat ice cream and cookies.

Kyli Chu: Kyli spends her time trying to finish the endless art projects she's lined up for herself, sneaking in book time whenever she can, and enjoying time with her family and friends. She has recently started acting and singing and still tries to find time in her busy schedule to write, babysit, and bake. After school, she either works with kids between the ages of three months and three years or plays ultimate frisbee.

Pia Apurva: Pia loves sailing, tap dancing, and debating. In her free time, she enjoys watching shows and spending time with her dog, Bala. Additionally, Pia loves playing instruments and has played anything from the ukulele to the trumpet.

Serena Saleih: Serena loves volleyball, reading, and listening to music. A long car drive is one of her favorite things ever, as well as staying up late with her close friends and family. In her free time, she always wants to get extra practice at her volleyball club's gym and eat Cinnabon cinnamon rolls while watching TV shows with her sister.

Meet the Illustrator

Sadie Chou: When she's not creating art, Sadie loves to read, sing, and play volleyball. In her free time, she loves to watch movies and TV, especially when she can discuss entertainment with her friends. She also likes to bake and test out new recipes.

Meet the Editors

Kristen Gianaris: Kristen is an international educator, award-winning photographer, and passionate advocate for social justice. In addition to the United States, she has called Egypt, Morocco, Switzerland, Taiwan, and China "home." In her free time, she enjoys creating pressed flower art, learning new languages, and indulging in other creative pastimes.

Paula Araque: Paula is a teacher and historian, most interested in exploring oral Latin American histories. She is a Ph.D. student at New York University and an avid public transportation advocate. When she is not dedicating her entire life to her cat, Chía, you can find Paula reading a book under a tree at the park, baking, or traveling around the world.

Sameeksha Singh: Sameeksha can often be found freewriting, belting out the lyrics to a Taylor Swift song, or practicing for whatever musical she's currently performing in. She also enjoys watching TV and spending time with her friends. Her favorite genres include fantasy, mystery, romance, comedy, and adventure.